Salon Madness
"The Shady Side of Beauty"

By
Jan Glaz

Disclaimer

While the stories in this book are true, some names and identifying details have been changed to protect the privacy of the people involved. Historical markers appear in various chapters. Language, photos, etc., are presented for literary effect. This is creative non-fiction.

CHAPTERS

INTRODUCTION

The episodes you are about to read hail from the North side of Chicago, mainly the Lake Shore areas, and primarily private owned beauty establishments. I, your author/reporter, and former cosmetologist gathered this information because I planned long ago to write a book on the subject; an expose of the madness that surrounds the Cosmetology Industry.

Unscrupulous people are everywhere in all professions. The following chapters are a collection of such behaviors as uncovered through interviews during the days when cell phones and internet use were in their infancy. I promised to keep my contributors; many were fellow hairdressers, off the record. Names of people and places have been changed to protect privacy.

You would be surprised at the antics between hairdressers and salon owners. And between competitive stylists who are on the prowl to steal away a good tipping client or a procedure for a winning hair color, or a chance to create a stunning haircut. They stoop down and use unlawful tactics. I was told of secret recording devices and hidden cameras in the customer seating and back room areas. Hair shows are another field of nightmares.

My first hand experiences are nestled within the chapters of this book. I tried out the hairdresser career for a few years in the City of Chicago. Although I maintain my license (valuable to receive discounts when making personal purchases at beauty supply stores) I have no desire to ever earn a living again in that realm of insanity.

The based on fact incidents within Salon Madness are an expose inspired by truth. Readers must hold in mind that not every beauty salon is into sneaky deeds, but most are.

Prior to becoming a patron it's a good idea to have a referral from someone who has had a lengthy experience with the salon. And it's advisable, when your body and finances are involved, to trust and have faith in the owner/owners of a particular establishment, as well as your stylists. "Just Be Aware!"

UNDER SURVEILANCE:
Barbara

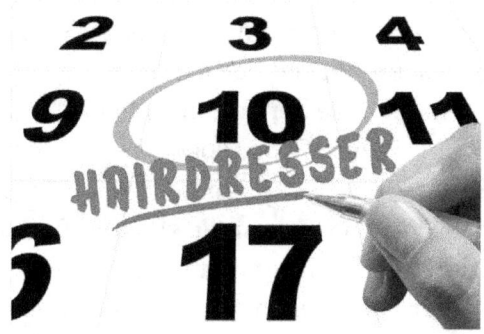

Barbara was a novice, fresh out of beauty school and no spring chicken. She was turning the 40th decade of her life. Barbara's fellow students in cosmetology classes were primarily late teens, early twenties, making her a misfit. She couldn't wait to graduate into an adult world and was anxious to tackle her profession. Like most newbies she was reduced to launching her career at a discount type of establishment, they advertise haircuts as low as $6.00 and other services at equally sliced margins. No matter, Barbara was overjoyed, she needed experience. So, tools in hand she arrived at the salon eager to learn.

On Barb's first day when she entered their arena carrying her plastic wheeler filled to the brim with hairstyling objects, her fellow stylists didn't bat a lash. She had just lugged the stuff up a steep stairwell attached to the back entrance, as it was uncouth to plod through the front area where the almighty customers were engaged in services. Barb parked her wears in a designated space by a row of lockers, as her new employee binder instructed. She dolly-upped her face and hair, straightened her outfit, and proceeded to enter the main room.

"Hello, my name is Barb, how do you do!"

That greeting fell on deaf minds. None of the other hairdressers looked up from their stations, so Barb strolled forward and soon noticed her name sticky noted to a salon mirror. This was to be her station; she was to take command of a small 5 by 5 plot of floor space. Before Barbara could set up her station, Greta, a veteran hairdresser and day manager approached. With a steely smile she told Barbara to please stop what she was doing and immediately remove the towels from the dryer, fold them and stack some above the wash bowls and others in cabinets. Greta pointed her fingers around the shop as she distributed her please orders.

"Oh, and when you've finished them, please clear the product shelves, dust the products and wipe down the shelves and reorganize the merchandise, and then please refill any low shampoo and moisturizer containers, and please Barbara, clean and sanitize both washrooms. "

Barb's first day passed without one single client, no tips and a meager $3.50 per hour pay rate. The next day she had an opportunity to service a few walk-in clients; one requested a facial, one a manicure and the other was a mom, her son required a buzz cut. The days passed with Greta making sure she spent most of her shift doing salon chores.

The veteran stylists were woman who had jumped from beauty school and into this entry level salon and stayed there for decades, primarily because they loved the power it gave their ego, and because each had grown a cache of regular clients, accumulated over stretches of time. Their favorite clients were used to paying low tips for low priced services. These veteran stylists were mentally stunted in one respect. Barb noticed they were addicted to lording commands and she was told that they belittled all and any newly licensed cosmetologists that crossed their path. Barb would soon to discover that a few of her fellow hairdressers were also addicted to illegal drugs and the bounties therein.

The owner of the salon rarely made an appearance; he arrived once a week, if the staff were unlucky. This older man had a business license on the wall that was in someone else's name. He was not a licensed cosmetologist, nor was he a U.S. citizen, he was a Canadian citizen. (You can own a salon without a Cosmetology license, but cannot perform a client service). He was a fellow who went by one name, Jack. When Jack was in the shop he sat by the register to collect dough. He made himself useful by screaming nonsensical orders at his workers. Unlike Greta, the word please, was absent from his vocabulary.

The shop was like a bad crime movie, not only towels, but money was being laundered within its walls. Barb failed to uncover the true purpose of the salon until one sunny and cloudy day when the shop was raided. Dear Greta was hauled away for selling drugs to a host of addicts disguised as clientele. Greta's drug deals had been captured on film in between highlighting, shampooing and hair cutting.

Barbara stashed away a heap of negative experience before the final curtain fell, before the washer, dryer and salon doors were permanently sealed. After Greta was arrested she accidently spilled her illegal activities to a gossip-go-round via a friend that worked in another salon, that friend broke Greta's confidence and passed Greta's shame to a bevy of other hairdressers, and they in turn, kept the story alive. The news Greta shared to that one friend came from the mouth of an undercover agent. He told Greta that authorities had rigged the shop with surveillance apparatus, hidden cameras, and microphones.

Newbie Barbara recalled that she had actually seen one deal transpire, though at the time did not connect it to drug activity. While Greta's client had his suds-filled head hanging backward into the sink, Greta slid a packet into one of his hands, and then as she helped the man from the wash basin she slipped her hand under his protective cape and nonchalantly secured a fistful of easily earned cash. At the time Barb thought it was a strange way to collect a tip. Shockingly, almost all Greta's indiscretions, over a period of a year, had been caught on camera!

Barb later found out that the salon's water massage bed and tanning booths had been primed for crime. Not only drugs, but sometimes during business hours sexual favors were exchanged for profit. Greta confessed to a pal that some evenings, after hours, she had participated in photo shoots, models were brought in for porno sessions; the results were shipped overseas.

Three veteran employees were arrested for criminal activity. The shop closed down, the owner disappeared, and Barb and other innocent hairdressers dispersed into new jobs. Eventually they all lost touch with each other. It would have been neat to know if these employees ever worked again at any type of money laundering drug dealing shops, but that fact is as secret, as secrets go.

The Back Room

Now if you believe in justice and accountability for one's actions and if you believe sooner or later thieves are caught then you will relish this expose. Talk about underhanded tactics transpiring at dishonest salons. The following example proves mindboggling corruption can occur in any form.

At one high end salon that shall remain nameless, the manager who had keys and was in charge of opening and locking the business woke up one night around 2 a.m. Her mind had split her pleasant dream open, to open doors: Her name, Beth.

Beth was having personal problems; she was estranged from her husband and was in the midst of divorce proceedings, she was facing a legal battle for custody of their daughter, who at the time was living with her husband's parents. Beth had received a subpoena on the day, of the night she uncovered a crime. Because her mind was upset she made mistakes that day with hair coloring and cutting. She was thankful when she finished her hours and closed the salon. But did she? Did she set the alarm?

When she sprang from a deep sleep to question herself she could not fall back to sleep, so she decided to dress and drive to the Salon to double check all the doors, and make sure the alarm was on. Beth parked her car in front, instead of the rear where employees are told to park, and then she climbed the stairs and opened the Salon. Beth hurried over to the alarm box to enter a code to deactivate it, if it were on. She was shocked! The alarm had not been set. Her subconscious mind alerted her to wake up, it was a miraculous feeling. Just as she had that thought she became frightened, she heard tinkering in the back where supplies were stored.

Beth's first reaction was to escape, alarm on or not, but being paid a higher wage as manager she mustered her courage and tippy toed around the beauty stations, she hugged the wall closest to the door leading into the supply room, where the sinks, washer and dryer were.

What a relief, it was the owner! At almost 3 a.m. in the morning.

"Mike, what are doing here, couldn't you sleep? I came down because I wasn't sure I set the alarm."

Mike was dumfounded, he didn't answer. In one hand was a large funnel and in the other a gallon container of an expensive product. These were used on the salon floor, clients paid bigger bucks to be shampooed and moisturized with well-known brands. On the counter next to Mike was a row of other containers. Beth recognized them as the shampoo and moisturizers usually found at discount stores. Mike was caught soapy handed.

He handled the stock, the ordering and delivering of supplies and kept all the invoices. The expensive products used on the floor had different grades, like volumizing, humidity-resistant, or ultra-shine. It was obvious he was pouring one grade of horrible cheap shampoo and moisturizer into containers with defining brand labels. A switcheroo!

Beth said, "What you're doing is against the law!"

Mike yelled back, "This goes on all the time. Grow up!"

Everything made sense the moment he said that. Beth and the other stylists were told never to throw away product containers after use but to save them to a large drum that belonged to Mike. That's where they dumped empty jars or bottles. When asked why, Mike grudgingly answered that he had to sort through the empties, as some manufacturers or suppliers ran promotions. That paid a bonus or gave discounts when containers were sent back. It seemed weird, but he was the boss. Beth realized that he might have been hauling a certain amount of empties home and filling them with something else, either to use at the salon or to ship back as unused.

Mike looked her in the eye, his voice lowered into threat mode, "I suggest you keep what you saw to yourself: Business as usual." He turned away from her to finish his dastardly deed. "Oh, and you did set the alarm, thank you for being so conscientious. When was the last time I gave you a raise?"

Beth's mind was reeling, she couldn't afford to lose her job, especially now. Mike was sure to put up a fight, a he said, she said. Because she was employed there for so many years as her taxes would indicate, if she applied for new employment she would have to list Mike's Salon on her resume. This meant his name would be listed on her job application. Mike, being the criminal he was, wouldn't hesitate to lie about her.

"Don't worry Mike. I won't turn you in, theirs a higher power in charge of all our actions and you will be held accountable." Beth turned and left the Salon. She was determined to secure another job after her legal battles, and she was certain Mike would give her a glowing recommendation. And then, Beth thought, 'I'll report Mike to the authorities, no matter how long it takes, I'm certain he'll still be playing in the back room'.

Many proprietors are never caught because reporting the escapades would cause tattler trouble and even legal expense to prove. Certainly, there has to be a number of salons that have been tattled on by former employees and they may have paid the price of cheating but only if their crimes could be proven without a reasonable doubt.

BEWARE OF THE STYLIST

Ego's run rampant in hair salons. The fighting and backstabbing is on the scale of an all-out war zone. Put the wrong personalities side by side, chair by chair, and a strategy to destroy each other is set into full swing. Sally was one of Joan's victims. Joan had the best, as they say in the industry, 'Chair' in the house. The chair is the hairdressers private work station the seat the client relaxes into, the chair faces the mirror, enabling a client to praise or complain about what he/she is paying for. The best chair is usually located in the front of the salon and has the most visibility.

It was Sally's misfortune to have transferred from her pleasant salon to one further from home, and to be assigned a chair with Joan's station, to her left. The previous hairdresser occupying that position had a low abuse threshold; she lasted about 3 months. Dear Joan was certain she invented hairdressing and would watch in the mirror, to her left and to her right any stylist watching her. She did this when performing what she believed to be her award winning services on a client. Joan's eyes had expert capabilities to both service her client and catch her fellows spying on her. If Joan caught someone, she wasn't ladylike, even if she had a client in the chair, her voice would escalate, "I saw you watching me, and how many times do I have to tell all of you to keep your eyes off me!"

Joan was very protective when it came to men's haircuts, because she had devised a blending procedure that garnished good tips. It was meant to be confusing. Changing clipper guard sizes back and forth, implementing comb over clippers and scissor over comb techniques. Like an artist, she could cut patterns such as tight edged lightning bolts, or star shapes, half-moon's, etc. into men and boy's semi-shaved heads. Intricate formal up do's that women wore to fancy occasions was another skill she guarded with a threat of physical violence if you dared to observe.

Reason being, Joan spent her free hours at home with her notebook and collection of dummy dolls (mannequin's students and professionals purchase either, male or female heads, you impale on a vise devise). Joan's habit was broadcast after a guy hairdresser had the misfortune of returning a pair sheers Joan had lost. From the moment the scissors went missing to the time she left the shop, she kept breaking into rants. Joan was positive one of the 8 stylist's on duty had stolen them. Because, as Joan reasoned, it occurred after she returned from the bathroom.

"Who's the thief?" She accused everyone, but kept looking at Sally. "Do I have to carry all my equipment with me when I use the John?" Joan's eyes again, never left Sally.

"I didn't take them, stop staring at me," shouted Sally.

"Why do you think that, are you guilty? You're the one closest to my stuff!"

"Take that back," Sally threatened.

"I won't press charges, just return them."

Sally lunged toward Joan but stopped midway and ran into the bathroom. Sally's abandoned client sat silent, afraid to add her opinion. And it didn't stop there, Joan called the owner of the salon and left a voice mail to report a theft, she wanted to get a search warrant and to not allow anyone to leave the shop. No one would oblige Joan, in fact a stylist who had opened the shop left without incident.

Throughout the entire scene, Joan paid no mind to the horrified customers having their hair cut, colored, styled or their nails glimmered. To ease the mounting tension, a few clients began searching for the missing scissors, as did a few stylists, but to no avail.

Joan began real tears, stressing to everyone forced to listen to her, how long she had saved up for the state of the art detailing sheers, and how she had just purchased them for $450 at the cosmetology convention the past weekend. After peddling her woe, Joan suddenly began cursing at fever pitch, and then flung a disinfectant jar holding combs and brushes off the top of her station. When it hit the floor, the solution splashed in the air. Maggie, a usually laid back stylist, hurried to the back room for a mop. The heavy glass jar splintered into large dangerous chunks. In the midst of rage, Joan packed her tool bag and stormed out of the salon.

A stunned walk-in customer, who would never walk-in again, sat at Joan's station with drippy black hair color oozing over her forehead and down the sides of her face. The fluffy cotton curbs that Joan had placed around the client's hair line were no longer fluffy. Sally stepped up to the plate and came to the woman's rescue. She apologized for the outburst, cleaned the woman's skin and installed fresh curbs. Kind hearted Sally, the accused, completed services on both her client and Joan's.

Christian, a guy stylist, was scheduled for the evening shift that day. Evenings had an add-on duty of sweeping and vacuuming, before locking up. This week it was Christian's turn. Joan was very fortunate that it was. Christian is a male equipped with keen observation. His mom or someone special must have taught him how to super-clean any area known to man or beast.

As he was sprucing the shop, Christian bent down to pick up a stubborn bobby pin that happened to be the same shade as the floor. They are hard to see unless you have been raised the way Christian was, Christian could spot a spot inside a spot. At each stylist station is a mirror, under the mirror is a counter, and the counter is supported by heavy legs with decorative foot ends. Unbelievable! Christian spotted the tippy, tip silver point of a scissor, like a fraction of a fraction of an inch. He used his muscle power to push the counter and then with the toe of his shoe, he kicked the tippy, tip object out of hiding.

Later it was determined that a sliver of space exists beneath every station counter's feet. Just enough tininess for a tiny object to slither into, but it had to be 'slitherable'. As soon as possible after the scissor rescue, Christian found Joan's phone number in the appointment book and buzzed her with his triumphant news! She asked him to come by immediately as she was booked early in the morning and would like to use her expensive new scissors. No mention of a reward, as Christian later related.

A few days after the incident, Christian was scheduled to work for Joan, as it was her day off. Before the shop opened, Christian gathered everyone together to blast forth a piece of Joan's private life. His tale set off a rage of hysterics. One young hairstylist yelled, "Joan's ticked in the head, she needs professional help... immediately. She should be fired!" Of course shop owners rarely if ever fire a stylist with a good following and with sales ability to push the salons thousands of items. This meant Joan could take her nuttiness to extremes and receive nothing but a warning from the boss.

"I rang her door bell," Christian began. "I rang, and rang and rang again. I pounded on the windows. Nothing helped. I circled around the house, opened a gate and crept up the back porch stairs. It was then my eye caught a shad of light between the window and the drawn shade. In that beam stood Joan, like a mad hatter, she was spinning a row of dummy heads, one dummy head this way and one that. Some had foils with splashes of hair color dripping onto the dummy's plastic face. Joan had shielded her floor with heavy tarps. I thought, this room must be her insane asylum. Music was playing and she thought she was singing opera but it tore your eardrums like a fire siren. In front of her was a large blackboard, I watched her race over with an eraser and in a tantrum, she pounded across her previous writing. I figured whatever she was concocting in her hair laboratory that night wasn't cooperating. When she left my eye range, I picked a fire log from a pile she had on the porch. I banged it on the back door that was attached to her asylum.

Without warning the door flung open. She was all sweaty, and she didn't ask me to step inside, instead she held out her hand, anticipating her sheers. I pulled the prize from my pocket and as soon as they emerged she clenched her palm around them in a tight squeeze. It was like she was saying to the scissors, "You will never leave my clutches again." Then her thin lips parted and shaped a faint thank you, followed with a brisk, "Have a good night". Boom! Joan slammed the door, and my reply, "You too Joan" hit the doors surface."

HAIR SHOW TRAGEDIES
Sneaky Joan

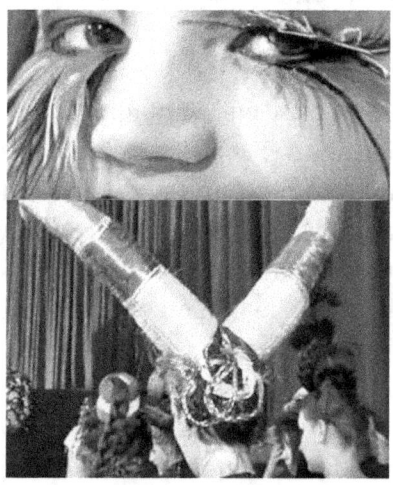

The young woman on the cover of Salon Madness represents a style that projects a specific mood. The model radiates defiance, as shown by the cut, color and styling of her hair. The latest styles debut at hair shows. It's well known that the most diehard hairdressers are also diehard competitors. They never miss trade shows. The spectacles encountered at Beauty Show Conventions, Cosmetology Expos or any and all manner of affairs presented within the beauty industry can at times be labeled 'Halloweeny'.

The chapter images shown above are an example. They characterize the outlandish that can be had at these events, and for a good cause. Besides the chance to become name-famous, which can lead to securing a sponsor and opening your own brand of products, or your own brand of salons, competitors are eligible to win other prizes. The awards offered by the circuses might pull in a year's supply of expensive wares, bounties that include anything and everything related to beauty services.

Joan, the maniac professional profiled in the previous chapter became addicted to hair shows because she believed it was only a matter of time before she would strike it BIG. Joan would brew up hair, facial and body products in her home laboratory; they were not approved by the Food and Drug Administration (FDA). Joan didn't care. One day she brought samples to the shop, a creamy aid to brighten your skin to appear teen age fresh. No one was willing to try it. So she packed it away and later presented the samples at that year's beauty expo. She had invested her savings and took out loans to pay for smart packaging, and for buy-ability, Joan's facial enhancer came with a money back guarantee.

At the expo Joan used herself to promote the age defying cream. Microphone in hand, she began to hawk her discovery in a booth she lined with humongous photos, before and after shots of men and women, people that had never used her lotion. Wow, sell she did! Not only did she sell every item she shipped to the extravaganza, she also collected a folder of future orders stemming from individuals and salons. In the end, Joan calculated her current and future profits would pay for the manufacture and marketing expenses she incurred. After breaking even, she imagined television advertising; magazines... the world would be her oyster. Joan was ecstatic, on the top of her game, nothing could stop her now! When she returned to the salon she treated the crew to a celebration outing of Pizza; all she could afford, until she whipped up another batch of serum.

Poor Joan, her success was short lived.

Before she could fill her creamy orders, she suffered a lawsuit. She was being sued for facial damages, and for life threatening allergic reactions that stemmed from unsatisfied customers who had eagerly smeared her product into their skin. These trusting souls not only wanted their money back, they wanted Joan, her house, car, and a chunk of any future earnings. Joan had bit into a nasty legal gig, lock, stock and barrel. Her salon mates later received word that Joan hired a lawyer; her defense would be in the realm of 'buyer-beware'. Joan insisted it was the customer's responsibility to inquire if the product met with FDA approval before purchasing it.

Jealous Lyla

Jealousy is a trademark that runs rampant during hair shows, sometimes to the point of sabotaging your competition. Lyla, a contestant, was caught leaving her rival's private booth after demolishing his born to win headpiece entry. Anyone who had the privilege of being shown the exotic creation, raved that hands down it had to win 1st place.

Hours before the judging, Lyla saw an opportunity to sneak into his cubicle; she had witnessed the owner of the piece having lunch with a group of people in the adjacent hotel restaurant. The coast seemed clear, so dear Lyla, sheers in hand, clipped the challenging headpiece to shreds. The floor was strewn with gobs of rare imported feathers that had been sprayed with splashes of neon and thousands of sparkling sequins sewn into patterns, fit to dazzle under any light, had scattered in the air and landed on the dummy head like rice thrown at a bride. It had taken her rival a chunk of cash and hours of skill and imagination to assemble and just minutes to destroy. Ms. Lyla never apologized; she displayed no shame or guilt. After the victim was notified of the death of his entry he began hyperventilating and had to be transported to a hospital. A doctor diagnosed his condition as a severe panic attack, administered tranquilizers and sent him on his way. Lyla ended up barred from all future events.

Comrades of Style

Another horrific sabotage case involved team presenters. "The Comrades of Style", a flashy team, had improved their techniques year by year, and always placed 2nd or 3rd. Rumors were flying that this would be the Comrades year as some teams had retired and the competition appeared weak; it was considered a shoe-in. Each Comrade member contributed their creative genius in an effort to snag the grand prize, consisting of thousands of dollars, a crown, and a commercial contract with an agency that promised fame and fortune. It was to die for; however a Judas walked among them. One of their crew members accepted a hefty bribe. He figured, as he said later, "Hey, there was no guarantee we would win. I had a sure thing, money upfront, I took it."

The Comrade's trader began trading a few months before the anticipated event. The spy busied himself with transporting the team's innovations to his benefactors. He handed over music scores, dance routines, and even the super-secret finale. The team that paid him, "Nuclear Brilliance" won the grand prize, the Comrades of Style, washed out. About a year later, as luck would have it, a loose mouthed girl swigging down shots of booze and ingesting amphetamines, began bragging. She not only spilled the incident she also named the Comrades traitor, "All's fair in love and war," said she, "Nuclear Brilliance" was engaged in a war to win... and we did."

ABNORMAL NORMAL CLIENTS
Bridget and Ken

Many years ago while spring cleaning my by apartment I found myself rummaging through old notes, and taped phone recordings. I compiled the following occurrences as the most interesting of the lot and stashed other incidents for future use.

Eccentric types exist all over the world, but Los Angeles, New York, and Chicago attract them at an accelerated pace. They're the artsy, creative, successful folk, business and political moguls and some average middle class wannabes.

Bridget and her husband Ken owned a fancy spa/salon along the lake coast area of Chicago, advertised as the Mag Mile shopping district. I've known Bridget since high school and was thrilled when she married a well to do gentlemen named Ken. Bridget agreed to my writing up the stranger than fiction cases of their normal, abnormal clientele. Our exchanges took place either by phone, as we were great chatting buddies, or on special occasions and get-togethers. Bridget and Ken have since retired and a clothing store occupies the once bustling beauty Mecca, but their experiences live on.

Their salon/spa was comprised of two levels; its square footage was off the charts compared to surrounding salons. I'll rename it for the sake of privacy "Heavenly Body Spa". Mind you some of your wealthiest people are the stingiest. Bridget said that she had price fights with almost all of their clients at one time or another. "Penny pincher braggarts," was one of Ken's favorite client nicknames.

One of the mainstay arguments that always popped up was a client insisting that a trim should cost less than a haircut. 'NO' the staff would counter; timewise and workwise they still had to go through the entire head: only cut off shorter amounts. Men with thin hair or semi bald fringe circling their heads would insist on a discount, because they figured they had less hair than Tarzan types. 'NO' said the staff. It was not the salons fault if you had less hair. Many children had more hair than adults, yes, they had to pay full price. And a child pedicure? They had 10 toes, no reduction because toes were smaller.

Besides penny pinchers, the Heavenly Body Spa drew in its share of bossy unreasonable patrons. If Ms. Paula ever knew that Bridget and her gang of employees at the spa were gossiping about her, she would have sued Heavenly Body in a wink of one of her false eyelashes. Paula, an elite wife of a real estate kingpin had nothing to do but shop and start trouble. Every so many months she had her hair trimmed. This client sometimes made an appointment and sometimes not. She would just drop in. Nevertheless, Heavenly Body always made time and space for her needs. Paula dressed to the hilt in silk, satin and jewels popped into Heavenly one afternoon, to complain.

"A few months ago one of your girls ruined my hair," she told Bridget. "I don't ever want her to touch me again."

"What was her name?" asked Bridget

"I don't remember, that's your job, look it up in your sales book?"

"Well, is she on the floor today, do you see her?"

Paula screamed like a banshee, "I just told you, can't you hear, can't you understand English, can't you just do what I ask? I don't remember faces of people who don't interest me. Just look it up."

"I'm sorry Paula, I'll be right back."

Well it turns out the stylist who cut Paula's hair the last visit had cut it the visit before that, and the visit before that. In fact Paula had requested her twice.

Bridget went back to Paula, but didn't badger her about being a numbskull.

"The stylist for your last session was Sylvia," Bridget said.

"Sylvia? Sylvia's one of my favorites! Are you certain?"

"I can show you if you want to see the log."

"If I wanted to see the log, I would have. I told you that's your job."

"Well Paula, Sylvia's name is logged in next to your name."

"Is Sylvia here today?"

"Yes, she's upstairs, but I'll have Noreen give you a trim, since you weren't pleased with Sylvia at your last visit."

"I don't recall the name Noreen?"

Bridget paged Noreen, and introduced her to Paula. Paula immediately became upset and instead of greeting Noreen, she blurted out, "I saw you on the floor a few months ago. You gave an older woman a haircut. When she left your chair I told myself to never have that beautician cut my hair. I'm sorry Noreen, but when the old woman left, she had half the hair she came in with, almost bald! You must have overused your thinning shears. Every strand of hair is a precious commodity when we age."

Paula turned to Bridget and asked, "Can you have Sylvia give me a trim?"

A Naked Dilemma

The next incident I'm willing to share is the most outlandish. It happened around 11:00 a.m. on sunny spring day. A gentleman entered the salon as a walk-in and said he desperately needed to tan himself. The tanning beds were open so the receptionist gave him a large towel, some protective glasses and ointment. The man entered. About 10 minutes later, he flew out of the room stark naked.

"The bed's on fire, help... help!"

He ran past everyone in the salon and streaked his naked body out the front door and onto the busy sidewalk. Patrons were aghast, they rushed over to the salon windows, they could hear him yelling, "Call the fire department, call 911, hurry, people are burning alive!" It was a sad hilarity to see pedestrians, cars and buses catch sight of him. The receptionist immediately called Police and within minutes they grabbed the guy, handcuffed him and stuffed him in the back of the squad.

Later in the day a policeman came into the salon to question the receptionist, Kim, and to fill out an incident report. The cop said the naked guy was higher than a kite. He passed out before they could take him to the station, so the officers rushed him, still dressed in his birthday suit, to the nearest emergency room where doctors saved his life from a drug overdose. The receptionist reached under the desk and handed over the man's clothes.

"Please tell him his tanning session is on the house, and there's no need for him to ever return."

Sara's Misfortune

The episode I'm about to relate is responsible for the demise of a young cosmetologist's career. Sara's misfortune was told to me by Ron. Ron's family owned a string of salons sprinkled throughout the suburbs of Chicago. Sara, now in her late twenties, became friends with Ron in high school, after which she managed to land a cozy paying job as a receptionist for a popular optometrist. But Sara loathed the work and felt creatively unfulfilled. Whenever Ron visited Sara he noticed that she was constantly buying hair and fashion magazines. Sara's home was overflowing with someone else's creative ideas.

"You can make good money, if you're good," Ron suggested, as she was flipping into the latest issue of Hair Styles."

"I have tossed the idea around, but don't think I can swing my job and school and besides the cost can range from $5,000 on the low end, to $20,000 or more for a high ranked school. It's like studying for a college degree. I talked with my tax and financial advisor and he said the majority of stylists earn no more than a waitress."

"He's right," Ron agreed. "The trick to big money is promoting yourself, to gather a following of clients that will follow you, even if you switch salons. It's up to you, your talent and your desire."

Sara was engaged to be married to a divorce attorney. Ron told her she didn't need to sit all day at a job she couldn't stand and that her fiancé Mark could help with tuition. "That's the way husbands are, they love when wifey is happy."

About a month after the discussion with Ron, Sara had a big blowout with her boss, Mary. The eye doctor accused her of messing up appointment schedules and forgetting to reorder supplies. Unfortunately, during their doomsday argument, Mary slammed her clipboard on Sara's desk and yelled insults.

"Week by week, Sara, your performance has been slipping, your mind is somewhere on another planet, and customers are complaining about your attitude. If you don't shape up, you'll have to ship out!"

Sara resigned immediately, and vowed to make a real go at marketing herself within the beauty industry.

Three quarters down the road to graduation Sara's life took a severe downturn. The lawyer boyfriend called it quits. It seems Mark had a previous wife and child, and they decided to get back together.

Her once bright future became an unbearable present day nightmare. Sara called Ron and begged him to lend her the money to pay what was left of her tuition. "I can work the loan off at your Salon; pay a percentage every month," Sara offered.

Ron and Sara were not close friends; they were more like friendly acquaintances. Ron told her that it was a pretty big chunk of change. He would need her to sign papers for the loan but it would be interest free. Sara couldn't do better than that, so she signed.

After graduation Sara's first few months employed at Ron's salon passed quietly. So quiet that only one person she serviced requested her a second time. Sara began questioning her choice of career, she began to hate it, but she owed Ron and was willing to bear the strain until she paid up; it was the right thing to do.

Little did Sara realize the consequence of that decision, and in hindsight she should have quit. If she had not decided to beat a dead horse she could have saved Ron from the stress of a lawsuit.

Regular clients are bearable, even fun and family like, but the characters known as one-timers, walk-ins, are a variety pack. They demonstrate zero loyalty and could care less about the proprietor and in many cases, they hope something will occur that enables them to take advantage of a situation. Like bad karma, a male in his thirties, complete with luggage, walked into Ron's establishment. After all, Ron had posted signs in the window and on the Salon door: "WALK INS WELCOME".

Sara was next on the roster to accept a walk-in. Stylists see it as an opportunity because a satisfied walk-in can morph into a regular gig. The man smiled at Sara and told her that he had just flown in from Florida and on the way to his hotel he spotted their Welcome Sign. Sara noticed the gentleman had bushy curly hair: Always challenging.

The client said, "I don't want my hair any shorter, I just want to spruce it up, clean the neck and ear area and even out straggling outgrowth. I'm in town for an important job interview, one that I've been trying clinch for years; it's scheduled for tomorrow morning."

He was very excited and wanted to belt out his career plans. Sara's first mistake that day was to participate in chit chat. A veteran stylist avoids distraction like the plague. Sara began to converse back and forth and while they were jabbering, she chose her largest clipper guard; it removes the least amount of hair.

The male in her mirror had a joyful grin plastered on his face as Sara attached the guard to the clipper. Grinning back, she switched on the motor, and while it was running, paused to answer a question he asked her about Chicago, and then, still talking, she bent down to adjust his chair and twist it into a better angle without realizing the clipper guard made contact with the chair and slipped off. Still chatting, Sara plowed into his hair. In one swift stroke she mowed a 2" wide path up the side of his head: Without a guard, it shaves to bald.

PANDOMANIUM! He freaked crazy... Sara screamed and ran to the back of the salon, where she literally collapsed on the floor. Sara was shaking like a leaf reported Gregory, the beautician who ran after her. The other stylists rushed over to confront the hysterical patron. Sara and Gregory could hear the man swearing and threating the shop owner, who was not present, with a lawsuit

In a fury, he yanked off his salon cape and scurried out the door. Accompanied by his newly scalped hair style, he dragged his luggage to the curb, and hailed a cab. Ron later told employees that the walk-in had to cancel his interview and had to have all his hair shaved off; it was his only option.

As promised, the client sued Ron for negligence, the cost of his trip, and his lost opportunity. Ron was fit to be tied, because the guy also tried suing for the amount of money he stood to make, had he been hired for the new position. Sara left the industry. Ron never talked to her again; he did however hold her to the loan contract, which she eventually paid off.

Crazed Caller

The craziness that goes on with customers is unending. This tidbit was told to me by a waitress, her regular hairdresser related it to her. Knowing that I was a licensed Cosmetologist she couldn't wait to add it to my expose. The waitress said: The owner of her neighborhood salon uses voice mail when they are too busy to answer the phone, one the hairdresser's haphazardly recorded this statement: Please leave a message we will return your call within the hour.

The recording played without a problem for near a year, and then one day the owner opened the salon and noticed the message indicator flashing. She pressed the play button. A female left her number and requested a return call. The owner dialed the number. A woman answered.

"You woke me up! Who is this? Oh, the salon! You lied on the machine; it's been hours since I left my message."

The owner checked the time of the call. The lady had phoned the shop at 3:00 o'clock in the morning. "You called at 3:00 a.m., the salon was closed, and no one was available to return your call."

The woman became irate. "So, you're saying it's my fault that no one was there? I will never patronize your establishment and I will make sure friends and family do likewise." She slammed the phone against the bedframe, blasting the owner's ear drum, and then hung up.

Needless to say the owner immediately amended the salon's recording. The new and improved message informed all callers, "We will return your call as soon as possible, during salon operating hours."

Beyond the Call of Duty

A female hairdresser, Linda, a person I did not know but soon would, was seated next to me at a wedding reception a few decades ago. We started exchanging weird salon tales. This happening happened during a hair coloring session at her shop. A client came in close to the end of the day, the salon closed at 9 p.m. and it was about 8:30 p.m. She insisted that she had to have her hair colored because an emergency had occurred and she booked a flight for the following evening. She was willing to pay a bit more and leave a generous tip.

The receptionist informed the woman that the time it would take to apply and process the color, wash it out and style it, would take about two hours and she did not want to accept the offer. The woman kept pleading and agreed to forgo a styling. "Just apply the color, wash it out, towel dry my hair, and I'll be on my way." The shop owner, Angela, who herself was an excellent cosmetologist and was managing the store that night, assigned one of the girls willing to stay on past closing. That stylist was Linda.

Poor Linda, the client had the equivalent of two heads of full hair, with various uneven coloring from previous adventures. She offered a choice of color and they both decided on the shade. Being a trooper, Linda dug right in but soon discovered that she could not even section the client's hair because it was all snarled and matted due to over processing. Linda used a whole container of cream softener before she was able to section and apply the color. It was after 10 p.m. when Linda set a timer to click off 40 minutes.

Meanwhile people kept driving up and knocking on the salon doors. The salon faced a busy street with a stop light and the public had an easy view while waiting at the red light. Linda wrote a couple of make shift signs, 'SHOP IS CLOSED", and placed them on the windows; to no avail. Cars periodically turned into the strip mall attracted by the shop's interior lights. The clock rang and finally, she walked her client to the wash basin.

Linda later confessed, "I was falling asleep on my feet, sweating from head to toe, nervous from listening to people trying to enter the salon. I couldn't wait to dry her hair and escort the unwanted client out the door. After I dried her hair, she walked to a mirror and had a conniption fit."

The client ran her hands through her hair and burst into tears, "I look ridiculous, the color is orangey, with pink and reddish streaks. This is not the nice mahogany we decided on. I can't leave looking like this, you'll have to do a color correction."

Linda went ballistic, "I'm not doing it over! I won't charge you, just leave!"

"I'm not leaving, and neither are you, fix it or call the police! "

Linda admitted to the woman that she did not have the experience to do a color correction.

"Then find someone who does, we are not leaving."

The client bolted her body next to the door and said, "Don't try escaping to the back exit either because I'll race you for it."

It was nearing midnight. The front door and parking lot were resting in peace. Someone else was sure to be resting too, Angela the shop owner. Linda knew that she was an expert in color correction and this lady had the worst botched head of colors Linda had ever witnessed. When she called Angela, the owner was shocked at the nerve of the client, protesting and staging a sit-in and said she would be right over. Angela lived about a half hour's drive from the salon. Linda could not leave the woman alone in the shop. They ended up in dead silence, watching T.V.

All of a sudden, the whole salon lit up. Two police cars were spinning into the parking lot. It was the topper for one of the worst nights in Linda's life. The police said a call came in that a possible burglary was in progress. As Linda was explaining the situation to police, Angela drove up. Things went from bad to worse. The police said Angela was breaking the law and they had to issue a citation. Evidently the town had an ordinance as to business hours for various businesses. The salon's business license was not approved for any work passed 9:30 p.m.

"Hey, gals do you know, it's like, 1:00 a.m.?" The officer asked.

The enraged client told the police she couldn't leave that she had botched hair. The policeman told the woman the shop is in violation, and they all had to leave, period. He added, "You can make a case against the business in small claims court and call the better business bureau to file a complaint against the owner, but right now you all have to leave."

The woman did file a complaint and that was about it. She did not have enough evidence to sue Linda for any misdeeds, besides it was hair. Hair grows away evidence. The moral of the story, said Linda, don't break your own rules, closing time, means closing time!

CLIENT VS CLIENT

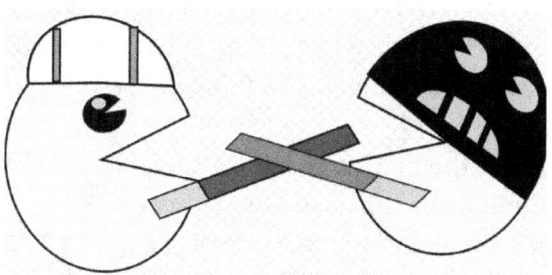

Racial Bigots

This book would not be complete without revealing the bouts that take form between clients. A popular salon is always overbooked. Within an atmosphere of all chairs filled, during all hours of a day conflicts between patrons abound. Some clients bond, though friendships that last the test of time are rare, battling clients are more the norm. Ann opened an establishment in a mid-income to low income neighborhood. Over the years it became the place to have your hair, fingernails, and pedicure serviced. Ann hired only friendly and patient employees.

Ann could not pick and choose her clients with the same skill. There are laws against discrimination. Her patron mix comprised of educated, semi-educated and non-educated people were akin to rubbing sticks together to start a fire. In fact Ann took a psychology course to gain insight on how to handle all the infighting.

One afternoon a young black girl became the butt of mean racial slurs. Two white teenagers conveniently exchanged black stereotyping in a voice loud enough for everyone in the salon to hear. Ann was outside checking on a delivery, the other hairdressers were taking care of clients. The white teens made fun of the type of hair styles black women wore, mocking their elaborated hair pieces and bandanas. One girl did her imitation of black slang language and then invented demeaning verses for a rap song. Both girls stood up, they swished their butts into wild African dance moves, occasionally tapping on a table to mimic drums.

When the black girl started to bawl, her stylist ran out to summon Ann. Ann asked the white chicks to leave immediately. They laughed; one of the girls screamed, "Call the police we're not leaven'." The other girl joined in, "Yeah, lady, haven't you heard of freedom of speech." Ann pointed to a sign on the wall that read, "We have the right to refuse service to anyone and to ask anyone to leave." Ann picked up the phone and waved it at the white girls. "You have one minute to grab your books and head out."

Non-Believer

Ann's Salon had a mix of faiths Jewish, Christian, Catholic, Muslim and atheists, etc. Never talk religion or politics in a mixed belief atmosphere. One mid-aged woman who frequented Ann's salon was an outspoken Born Again Christian named Lynette; her life mission was bent on saving souls, usually accomplishing God's work by scaring people. Lynette survived because most people ignored her advances, nicely.

"See the light of Jesus, or die in sin and suffer in darkness for eternity," Lynette preached.

It was annoying and Ann had pep talked her employees to hold their tongue and get through Lynette's occasional visits as quickly as possible. The reason Ann put up with this patron was because a congregation of Born Again Christians made up more than half of Ann's regular clientele; on

Lynette's recommendation. Saying good bye to Lynette would mean saying hello to loss.

Every other phrase in Lynette's normal conversation was related to Jesus and scripture. Always on the lookout, she managed to recruit souls at the slightest opportunity. Out from her pockets or purse popped heaps of Christian propaganda. Most of Ann's customers politely accepted the offerings. They produced a "thank you" even if they didn't mean it.

Unfortunately, an atheist had scheduled an appointment and was assigned the stylist next to the Holy Roller; Ann's name for Lynette. Within 5 minutes the whole salon went up for grabs. It was a busy Saturday afternoon. A wedding party had been booked. The bride and bridesmaids were positioned in front of mirrors watching their hair turn into eye popping up do's strung with jewels, ribbons and flowers. Other clients were having their hair colored and cut. Nail technicians were busy applying manicures and fancy nail ornaments to a long row of hands.

The atheist raised her voice, "Mankind invented God. Mankind wrote the bible and imagined the words came from the God they invented. People can imagine seeing ghosts or angels and they will see them. It's the way our brains are wired, healings and miracles occur for non-believers as often as believers, that's a fact!"

"Miracles happen to non-believers only by the grace and mercy of God!" shouted Lynette. "Satan is your bed fellow!" Lynette then quoted a verse from the bible and said, "I'll pray for you to see the light, as a Christian I have to pray for your salvation."

"You're the one who needs to see the light lady! You live in a fantasy world with other inmates like yourself. Your imaginary God put you in charge of saving my soul and other souls that don't belong to you? Mind your own business!"

The atheist and the Christian began screaming their beliefs so fast and furiously that no one could make out a word they were slinging. In a surprise move, the Christian jumped from her chair and struck her fist into the atheists jaw. The non-believer's head pitched backward and banged against the chairs metal frame. Ann intervened; she pushed Lynette away from her enemy. Two other stylists ran to Ann's defense because Lynette attempted to hit Ann.

Meanwhile the atheist was busy swearing and screaming at Lynette, "Assault and battery! Crazy Christian, I have witnesses!" A large lump had developed on the atheist's battered head and her pulverized face swelled double in size, the cheek that took the whack had blushed into a bluish black shade of ugly. When the atheist caught her damaged reflection in the mirror she became hysterical. "I'm heading to the police station right now, so they can take photos".

It was the last Lynette straw. Ann had no choice but to refuse future service to her Holy Roller, and to say "au revoir" to most of her business. The religious turmoil continued in a new setting, Lynette and her flock began frequenting a rival salon a few miles away from Ann's Shop.

Eavesdropper Drops

The meekest of them all may not be as meek as one would like to believe. The next case rising from my files of madness at the salon is an example of eavesdropping. These nosy individuals lurk in public settings and they may look as if they are paying zero attention to what people in their vicinity are saying or doing. Eavesdroppers will pretend to be reading, writing or to be engaged in activity. The professional eavesdropper will never look over and thereby alert a talker that they are being observed.

The worst of worst eavesdroppers do this deed almost hobby like, when they are feeling lonely, bored, or when they don't have a life and everyone else's is more interesting. They relish hearing others private business like an animal relishes a good meal. Ask Paul, he was the victim of a vicious female eavesdropper.

Paul always requested a beautician named Vera for his haircuts, and Vera was also my Aunt Adeline's hairdresser and it was my Aunt who relayed this shocker to me from beginning to end. Here's how it went down.

Paul visited beauty salons as opposed to barber shops because the salon's catered to both male and female patrons. As he tells it, it seemed more exciting and he liked watching females in various stages of beauty making. Paul mentioned to Vera that he met his 2nd wife at a beauty salon. "She was drop dead gorgeous. I was new to that salon and she was a long standing regular. When I heard that, I became a 'regular' too!" Paul added, "That salon closed and a coworker recommend this beauty shop."

Paul was quite a blabber mouth for a robust male. He had his hair buzzed every few weeks and as soon as he sat in the salon chair he began spilling out his private life. Vera said she felt like a priest hearing confession. "I had no choice but to listen, and it was embarrassing."

It so happened that this salon acquired a new client, Noreen, she was a seasoned snooper and whenever this busy body was lucky enough to have an appointment around the same time as Paul, it made her day. Paul tantalized his listeners with his marital bed episodes, his nasty in-laws and their constant bickering, and all their out and out fights. He easily talked about his salary, his taxes, his mortgage, his wife's first husband and the two unruly children she had with the man. To Noreen it was like living in a grand soap opera whenever he sat within her ear range.

On one not so sunny day Paul made a huge blunder, he mentioned his wife's maiden name. Noreen almost fell off her chair when she heard it. He also confessed to Vera that he was having an extramarital affair with the receptionist at the company he was employed with.

He acknowledged, "She's a chunky gal, not a looker, very reserved and proper until you take her to a motel room and lock the door, than she translates into the sexiest woman I've ever met."

Noreen happened to be a casual friend with someone who had the exact last name as Paul's wife, Julie. Noreen became hyper and cut her salon visit short so she could investigate what her prying ears had just heard. The eavesdropper couldn't wait to drop a possible marital bombshell.

As it turned out, the casual friend was a distant relative to Julie and had met Julie now and then on different occasions. Noreen excitedly spilled all Paul's beans to this relative, Sandra.

And then, some months later, Paul's wife Julie attended a baby shower. She was approached by Sandra who expressed her condolences.

"I hope you and your husband can work things out, I'm sure he loves you and not the other woman, from what I was told it's truly just a sexual fling."

Julie was flabbergasted, she could not believe her ears, she immediately left the baby shower and cried like a baby all the way home. As soon as Paul arrived home she confronted him. Paul would not admit to anything so Julie did some investigation on her own and discovered motel charges on his business account.

The very next day, she hired a lawyer and eventually, received a nice divorce settlement for her and her children.

When the intrusive Noreen heard from Sandra that the couple had divorced she proudly told Vera, "If it was not for me, that snake in the grass Paul would still be cheating and getting away with it." The cruel minded Noreen congratulated herself for she felt she had exposed a cheater and that she was a hero to be recognized, a doer of good deeds.

ICKY STOMACH TURNERS

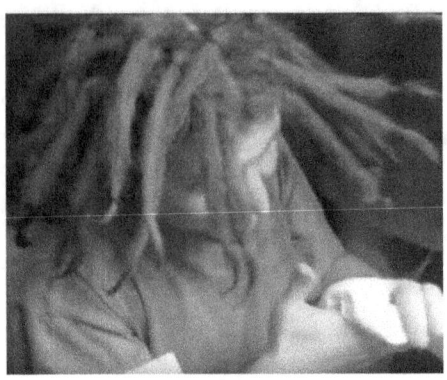

We can understand a doctor or a nurse dealing with professional stomach turners but most people don't associate the dutiful hair stylist with a list of repulsive human icky's. Rhonda one of my regular stylists who cut, bleached and styled my hair called me one day after I left her a message that I had decided to attend beauty school.

"You told me you would never study to be a nurse because you had a weak stomach. Well, before you venture further I have to warn you that you will encounter a host of stomach turning icky's".

Rhonda's warning sent me into yet another research project and what I discovered is revealed in this chapter. Another one of the reasons I cut my cosmetology career to the bone and left for greener fields.

First off let me introduce you to a male hairdresser, we'll call Scott. I jotted his story down on a table napkin during lunch. Years ago I wasn't as organized and I had an entire dresser filled with notes and my inspirational authoring ideas written on everything from napkins to torn-off pieces of cardboard once belonging to packaged goods like cereal boxes, even opened unwanted junk mail, almost any type of writable material I could grab hold of, worked for me.

Eventually, I very, very, slowly over the years organized my memorabilia. However, I was too lazy to rewrite hundreds of notes so I categorized them and shoved them into food storage bags for safe keeping. One category was labeled 'ICKY'. Scott's icky horrors sat waiting for publication at the bottom of my scrap journal. If you just ate please save most of this chapter after digestion.

An elderly woman client came in to have her hair styled for an important occasion. Scott cheerfully escorted the charming lady over to the wash basin, draped her and proceeded to shampoo. He hosed with warm water, added shampoo and without gloves, as many beauticians do not wear them for an average hair wash, he proceeded to scrub starting from the hairline back, and then from the nape of the neck to around the ears and sides of her head and then back again to the crown area. And then... that's when it happened!

Scott was so shocked he let out a belly scream, being a sensitive type of male might have had something to do with his escape into the back room. Scott was convulsing, trying to hold back vomit and rushing to clean his hands. The client bolted up from the bowl at sat innocently in her chair, as she watched the commotion. She had seen it before, it had happened at various salons now and then.

Here's what happened: Pieces of bloody scalp with hair follicles attached fell into Scott's hands, sticking to his fingers were nice sized chunks and tinier remnants. The salon staff approached the client just as she announced, "He'll be alright; my scalp must have peeled off."

Scott could not function and left the salon from the back exit immediately after disinfecting his hands. The lady said it was her medications and that it didn't happen very often. It usually happened when her doctor changed one ineffective medication and introduced another into her system.

The next event is a more common occurrence and I print it as a medium 'ick'. It's known as the head full of fleas or those nasty wee lice; scabies. It's bad in kids but especially hard to stomach when their found romping around adult heads. You would be surprised how many clients at discount hair shops walk in off the streets and ask for service, knowing they have itchy buggy heads of hair. It's definitely not widely publicized within the cosmetology field, so I decided to give it some play.

Take a second and please notice the photo at the top of this chapter. The hairstyle on the image of this gentleman is named; dreadlocks. They are very popular in our society for adult males, females and for children. People can wear them indefinitely; like to death do us part. People should use proper care and learn how to clean and moisturize this matted look or suffer the consequences.

The grossness I will now describe happened to an acquaintance who owned a barber shop. As he tells it a man came into his shop with dreadlocks that he had lived with for years. He wanted to start a new leaf in life. He told the barber he had recently registered for trade school and that he decided to have his entire head shaved clean. Classes did not start until the fall and his hair would have time to grow in.

The owner of the shop assembled his tools, caped the client and using his hands, began to assemble the dreadlocks in position for shearing, but as soon as the client's scalp met his eyes he backed off. What he was looking at was a discolored bluish-green scalp. It was baggy and loose. Crusty dried pus had accumulated throughout his dreaded scalp.

The owner asked the client, "When was the last time you cleaned your head?" The client professed, "Not sure, maybe four or five years. It's not really necessary with dreadlocks and that's why I like to wear them." The owner of the shop informed the man that he needed to seek medical help, the sooner the better. As the wannabe student was leaving his shop, dreadlocks in place, the owner suggested postponing school for at least six months.

In case my readers digestive tracks are flip flopping, I will end this chapter. But first, one more 'ICK', and it's a smelly one. Unkempt people many times are not aware of the fact that they are exuding an odor. Maybe they're suffering from illness, depression, live alone or because they are no longer part of a work force, they become lazy about hygiene.

Jackie was a friend of mine for a couple of years. She reported to me that at her salon a female arrived without an appointment. Her body odor was as potent as an aggravated skunk, if not worse. Thank goodness she was the first customer of the day. All the hairdressers visibly started to gag and one of them hurried into the supply room. When the stylist returned, she nonchalantly whizzed the entire salon with bathroom deodorizer.

The smelly woman became unhinged. Not for a second did she attribute the spray action to her presence. She immediately yelled at the girl sprayer. "What are you doing, are you crazy, do you want to asphyxiate me and everyone in this shop?" And then she added, "I'm going to report this to the EPA (Environmental protection Agency). Holding her nose closed, she briskly left the shop, never to be seen again!

SLOWPOKE ANNIE

I came across this mind boggler from the time I had attended Cosmetology School. It was related to one of my classes and a teacher named Ms. Pat. Prior to teaching she owned a shop she called her Beauty Castle, so Ms. Pat had plenty of first hand advice to pass on to her would be beauticians. This teacher was a stickler when it came to students finishing their projects on time; or sooner. She always emphasized time during every assignment. "We grade on time as well as skill," Ms. Pat would preach.

The way a cosmetology career takes off, once you graduate from Beauty College you have to pass a stringent exam set up by the State to obtain a license. Thus, to be eligible take a State exam you have to log a required number of graded hours from the school. Grades are given for book studies and practical procedures.

Students begin by practicing their skill on mannequins, then on each other, and then they're allowed to experiment on Guinee's. These are people who visit beauty schools and save mega money by having students conduct all types of salon services. The Guinee's don't seem to mind an occasional trip to the doctor or a trip home crying about a botched haircut, hair coloring, a nail, skin or scalp infection. In fact they sign a release prior to their service which is designed to protect the students and school from lawsuits, although the safeguard doesn't always pan out.

Aside from tuition, cosmetology colleges also sell products, thus they thrive financially from the revenue provided by Guinee's. There's a pecking order attached to the price a Guinee will pay. If they request a senior, a student who is near graduation level, the price is higher. If they accept a true novice still working on mannequins with plastic hands and feet, then the price of a service is adjusted down. The Guinee's are a valuable tool for students; the experience is likened to an internship whereas they face a variety of challenges and a heap of ostentatious human beings. A precursor to the pitfalls they will surely fall into. Students aren't paid but they can accept tips, and some Guinee's have paid their favorite student a nice hunk of dollars, so students compete in hopes of capturing a good Guinee as a regular.

As Ms. Pat stated, students are tested according to time as well as performance. If they cannot wrap a perm, create an up do, color hair, cut hair etc. within a prescribed amount of time it marks against their grade. The reason time peeved Ms. Pat to distraction could be traced back to a negative time experience that took place at her Beauty Castle Salon. Dear Ms. Pat never missed a chance to tell incoming students her tale of "Slowpoke Annie". I heard Ms. Pat tell it many times during the year I logged in my hours.

Annie, a seasoned stylist seeking a position, ventured into Ms. Pat's Beauty Castle Salon boasting that she had a readymade flow of clients. Of course Ms. Pat was delighted and accepted her right away. She even dismissed another beautician who was taking space in her salon and was not generating clientele or product sales.

As soon as the other stylist left, Annie parked in her space. Annie's clients, all of two, arrived for their scheduled appointments the following day.

"It was maddening to watch!" Ms. Pat would say. Annie moved in slow motion, but she only did this when she sat a client.

As an example, Ms. Pat stated the when Annie's appointment was seated, Annie would manually massage their scalp and then she would pick up a brush and ever so 'slowly' brush the client's hair, taking only a certain number of strands with each stroke, lifting them to brush them every which way. After brushing she would repeat the same procedure with a fine tooth comb. Annie had convinced people that by combing out individual strands in that manner it was healthy for their hair, bringing oils through the length of the hair shaft. As a result, any client that believed whatever Annie told them, would stay with Annie and Annie was certain they would never be able to demand from anyone else the kind of services they received from her.

But that was only the beginning. Ms. Pat said for no apparent reason everything she performed was 'slow'. Sectioning hair, lift and clamping hair, ever so slow shampoos, super slow haircuts, and mega slow color and styling. In other words, Annie stretched services to take from two to four times longer than average.

"I was fit to be tied after her first month at my salon," Ms. Pat told her students. "In an 8 hour work shift, Annie was lucky to finish 4 or 5 clients." For Ms. Pat this meant Annie's station was always filled and walk-ins had a longer than average wait and would walk out. Fewer customers meant fewer product sales. A chain reaction had been set in motion that soon spread like a virus to Ms. Pat's other stylists.

The other hairdressers noticed that Annie's clients, instead of dumping her for wasting their time, tipped her royally. Annie told her co-workers that her clients felt coddled and confident that Annie was doing a much better job than any other hairdressers. They were a strange brand of loyal customer.

To Ms. Pat's horror the other hairdressers began to try out Slowpoke Annie's routine. A few found clients that fell in love with slow, but most customers instead of feeling coddled felt irritated and complained to Ms. Pat.

Annie had managed to single handedly slow down the salon's operation. Less than 4 months after hiring, Ms. Pat nicely asked Slowpoke Annie to please take her entourage of clients to another salon. Ms. Pat reasoned that Annie was a wandering stylist planting her brood wherever she found a hungry shop owner willing to take them in.

After Annie left, Ms. Pat held a meeting with her employees and informed them that if they continued to act like Annie they could follow her right out of the shop. At the meeting one her employees stood up to Ms. Pat.

"It's wrong of you to stand over us with a clock, I never heard of such a thing. Working a bit slower works, there is a place for it and tips are better. Look how successful Annie is."

Ms. Pat answered, "This isn't a construction site, it's a business, my business, and if you slow builders want to build an empire, build it somewhere else!"

HANDS UP

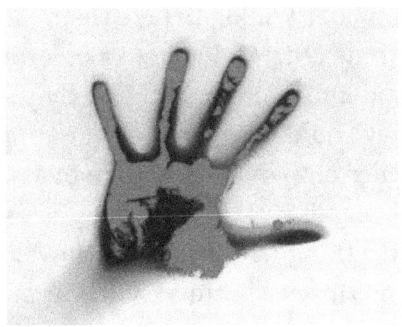

Dolly, they called her, Dolly. She was hired at a Salon on Clybourn Street, the Salon has long since vanished but the tragedy remains. I passed the exact corner when I revisited the area in 2012. The original structure had been torn down. Dolly was an attractive African American hairdresser. The owner, also African American, was gunned down after Salon hours. Dolly used to hang out at one of the Piano Bars located on Ontario Street. I believe it's still doing business as of 2015, the name of the place; Redhead Piano Bar.

I met Dolly around the Holiday's back in the day. I came in with a few of my hairstylist friends. Poor Dolly, this was the second time she was employed at a Salon that was targeted for a hold-up.

"All Salons are at risk during the holiday season," Dolly said. Although Dolly wasn't present when the owner was shot on Clybourn, she was present at her previous employment on the night a gunman came waltzing in near closing. Dolly said it was the most frightening event in her life.

The man must have been casing the salon. It was a well-known and well-advertised franchise still in business that shall remain nameless in this telling.

The rules in Dolly's employment manual stated that two or more employees must be in the Salon at closing; however the franchise owner cared less about enforcing that rule. Time and again he would appoint just one stylist to close the shop, to divvy up the credit and cash numbers for the day, and then drive down the street to the bank and deposit any cash in the overnight depository.

Dolly was always uncomfortable alone in the shop at closing and complained to the owner, who always would point his arthritic fingers at the exit. "You're free to quit anytime you like."

Dolly had a following, she was earning good money and the economy was not doing well. It had taken her near two years to build regular clients. It had taken her 6 months to secure the job at that franchise. At the time he hired her she was a newbie.

The employees knew the owner had his friends or relatives periodically spy on the stylists. One guy stylist was fired because the owner's friend came to the door a few minutes before closing and the guy scheduled to close that night told this would be customer that the salon was closed.

So when Dolly got wind of the traps the shop owner pulled she vowed to allow a late comer in, dangerous as it was. "You can be very stupid when you're new and hungry for work," Dolly told us at the piano bar.

As she was walking the man to her station for a haircut he grabbed her tightly around her waist using both his arms. She could hardly breathe. And then he put one of his big smelly hands over her mouth as he jammed her body, face first, against a wall.

"Put your hands up and on top of your head and don't move or it will be the last thing you ever do." He took his hand from her mouth and said, "One sound and I'll rape you before I stab little cuts all over your body."

51

Dolly started to tear up at the telling, "He took the edge of a jagged knife and ran it slowly down my cheek and stopped at my neck and shoved the point into my skin."

My friend reached over to hug Dolly, just as the piano man played a fitting tune. When Dolly stopped crying she continued. "I slumped to the floor from fright and curled my body in womb position. He found a towel and shoved part of it in my mouth and dragged me into the back. I was sure I was going to be raped and killed. He knocked me out and when I regained consciousness I was alone. My head was aching. I checked myself, I had not been raped."

Dolly said she wobbled to the phone and called the police. The man had taken all the money from the shop. She couldn't help the sketch artist because her mind began to block out the horror. When confronted the owner denied any wrong doing. He told authorities that Dolly should not have allowed anyone in because she was alone.

Dolly tried to make a case with the franchise and to enlist the help of the other employees to testify against the owner. Of course no one wanted to get involved. She quit, and without another job on her horizon none of her regulars followed. In fact, she had been warned by the owner that the clients she had accumulated belonged to his shop and he would bring a lawsuit against her.

MOVIE STARS & MODELS

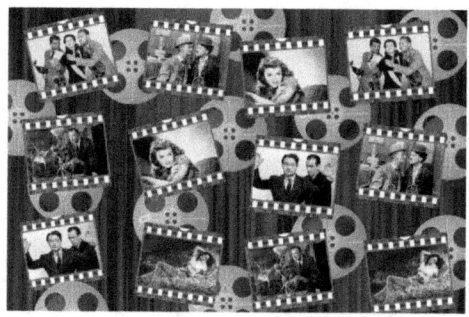

"Gimmie a Break!" this was Jaclyn's favorite expression. It originated from her exposure to a client trade constant. Every stylist at one time or another has encountered the movie star/model customer.

I can personally vouch for the experience. It happened to me countless of times throughout my mini-career as your local friendly hair stylist. I call it dealing with an undiagnosed mental illness, one that there's no antidote for and no prescription medicine as yet has been devised.

These mind boggling clients come into hair salons with a bevy of photos. Ok, sometimes just one, but most of the time a bevy. As soon as you're ready to service them, out comes a picture of their favorite movie star. The star could be a person who lived decades ago and is now dead. Sometimes the crazies pull out a photo from the morning edition of the local newspaper and relate to it. The worst is a photo of someone they despise in every way except the famed person's hairdo or savvy haircut.

Fashion models are huge; these photo arrivals are usually favored by women clientele. The heartache arrives when a photo is of the client themselves. In the photo they're in the young and virile stage of life. The hairstyle looks good because they do.

As luck would have it, one day Jaclyn and I simultaneously attracted people who spent their lives in fantasy land. My client was a man with an advanced case of balding. He whipped out a vintage picture.

. "Look, it still stands the test of time. My dad took this with one of the first Polaroid cameras on the market. The kind you had to rub a stabilizing stick over after you timed the chemicals that produced the image."

I glanced at the antique he handed me and squinted for all I was worth. Then I grabbed my magnify tool. I barely made out the image of a man, let alone his hair.

"Can you cut my hair like it is in the picture?"

"I can only see the front view," I answered.

"Well, if you can see the front then because you're a professional you must be able to determine the rest of the cut."

I carried the picture to our large windows at the front of the salon, magnifier in tow. It was then that I spotted a twenty something guy with a handsome face who wore his hair parted from the dead center of his forehead-zagged along the top of his head.

"I don't think you have enough hair for me to cut into this style," I gently told him.

"Sure I lost a bit of hair, but there's plenty left."

The man ran his finger through his thinning follicles.

Please Miss my grandchild is getting married and I don't want look my age. Color and cut it like the photo."

I began the color process and tried like heck to part what was left of his hair in a zig-zag.

He was not happy with the results and yelled, "I look like an idiot. I'm not paying for this!"

I told him I was sorry, but I had to charge for the hair color product and my time. "I did warn you that it was not possible and you insisted it could be done. Now you see it cannot."

The irate customer flung his old photo on the floor where I had cut his hair. "Sweep this up with my hair, now that you ruined me it's useless to take to anyone else. The wedding is this weekend."

He looked at Jaclyn, "I should have picked you instead of her. You're young."

He turned his aging face back to me and said, "You have old eyes, you couldn't even see the picture why did I think you could cut my style. I'll pay you only because it's my fault. When my hair grows back, I'll be sure to always have young people take care of me."

Jaclyn was still servicing her customer. The lady had brought a picture of a young model from a magazine. Not only that, she had put the photo in a frame and set it on Jaclyn's station so Jaclyn could keep her eyes on it as she worked.

Twenty minutes later everyone in the salon heard the women yell at Jaclyn, "Watch when I hold this photo next my face. I don't look anything like it."

The enraged customer then turned toward the other clients in the shop. She held the frame next to her face and to each person she said, "There's no resemblance, it's as if I didn't bother to bring in what I was asking for."

The model in the photo the client brought in clearly had extensions and hair pieces attached. And she had an entirely different shape of face than the customer.

Jaclyn calmly walked up to the lady and said, "Gimmie a break... you'll never look like the model in that picture, even if you have plastic surgery."

The lady was stunned at the remark and promptly huffed over to the front desk. She paid the receptionist, she didn't leave a tip, but she did leave an insult.

We all watched. She walked like a maniac and entered the service area pointing a finger at Jaclyn. Then as loud as possible she asked Jaclyn, "Who did you pay off to get your license? What did you do to get this job, sleep with the boss?" Photo frame in hand, Ms. Client left the salon with her favorite model, and was never seen again.

BODY DISASTERS 101

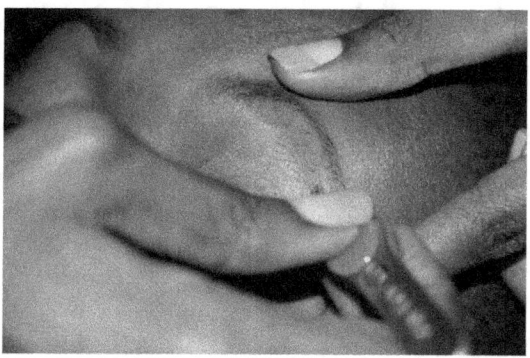

Let's not hear it for beauty school. Beauty classes are not beautiful and disaster is always lurking between the isles. Failed beauty victims and botched beauties rarely die but some feel they should. Read on and you will learn the truth of what I confess.

I ran into Rhonda, literally. I was at the mall and running late. I found a clearing and began jog stepping as fast as I could and that's when it happened, "Bam" smack dab into Rhonda's chest. She screamed and I screamed, and then we both recognized each other and shock faded into laughter.

Rhonda had to be in her 50's but she was a great camouflage artist. "Rhonda, I'm sorry I ran into you, no, I'm not sorry," I laughed again. "It's so wonderful to see you and you look terrific. I'm late for sure now, but let's have lunch sometime."

I pulled out my business card and then continued running.

About 3 weeks later I received a message from Rhonda and we set a date. Everything was going fine until her cell phone rang. I felt odd sitting there listening to her whisper secrets into her phone. When she hung up her face had lost its youthful glow.

Rhonda told me the call was from her brother, who owned a cosmetology school; his business license was being revoked and he was in deep legal trouble.

"Wow, that's drastic. What caused the action?"

"Not one, but two cases of sexually transmitted disease had been reported to the health department in connection with his students."

I had been munching on a bread stick when she dropped the sex bombshell. I started to gag and tried to talk at the same time.

"You can't be serious! Please share the details."

I pulled out my wee note pad.

"Rhonda, I save tidbits like these. Do you mind if I jot down what happened?"

"You can jot but if you tell anyone, don't ever use our names"

Our lunch arrived and Rhonda thought it best to eat first, in case I had a weak stomach. We chatted about our family and friends and caught up on years of experiences.

I tried eating as fast as I could, as I was anxious for all the low down on sex at school. Finally Rhonda pushed her chair forward along with her voice. I pushed my chair forward to meet her words.

I was mistaken, it was not a juicy sex tale, it was a clueless student who had no idea that when a rule states to throw away or sterilize items used on one client as not to use them on another, the rule had to be observed.

A young woman who came into the beauty school ended up with herpes on her face because the student applied wax using a stick she used previously to perform a Brazilian wax on a client.

"And the second, case?" I inquired.

Rhonda opened her cell phone to a text message and passed it over to me.

"This is what my brother texted last month; it's the name of the disease the doctors had to treat on another woman who suffered a similar fate."

"That's quite a coincidence, Rhonda." Is the school next to a strip club or unscrupulous massage parlor?" I glanced at the message, and then wrote a few notes.

The infection was molluscum contagiosum and it is transmitted through sexual contact. Rhonda said it was a highly contagious disease which is making the case against the school quite serious. The incidence happened due to an action known as 'double dipping'. The cosmetology student innocently used an unclean applicator, not realizing the previous service had been on a sexually corrupted female.

Before Rhonda left, we chatted about waxing. My tale was not near as spicy but when I attended school one of the girls in our class neglected to inquire whether her client used any type of medicinal treatment on her skin, before she engaged a waxing. Because of a medicinal the client had used on her face, the wax seared the clients skin causing severe burns that had to be treated by a doctor.

Important details somehow float right over a students head. It doesn't pay to save money and risk that one time mistake that can cause havoc to your body.

Before I graduated I had my personal share of mishaps. They occur when students are assigned to perform on other student, as practice.

A fellow student gave me a pedicure and I ended up with a toe infection on the large toe of my left foot . It was so severe, I could not wear my regulation school shoes.

About two months later, I contracted an allergy from some cheap product the school had us handle, and a few days later when a new student bleached my hair, it started to fall out of my head because she blobbed to much bleach on various sections and strands... and not enough on others.

I had to have a color correction for my remaining hair. I asked the teacher to administer it. Based on these incidents, I put in a request to the owner of the school to spare my body and release me from any further students in training.

I highly unrecommend taking your precious body, mind and spirit into a cosmetology school for a low cost salon service, unless you love to gamble: The stakes are high!

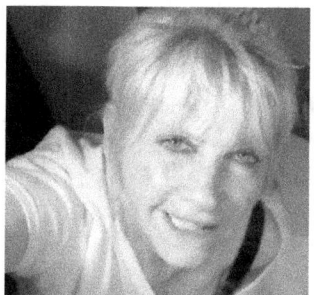

Thanks for Reading

From 2011 to 2022 author, Jan Glaz, was busy as a newspaper reporter writing front page stories for Village View Publications, Inc., located in the heart of downtown Chicago. Since 2016 she has successfully published and sold a wide range of best-selling, top reviewed, fiction and non-fiction books.

People who love a good read will love Jan's collection of best-selling Fiction and Non-Fiction books. For access to all currently published titles please visit:
amazon.com/author/janglaz

"Wonderful books are eternal, Jan strives for wonderful!"

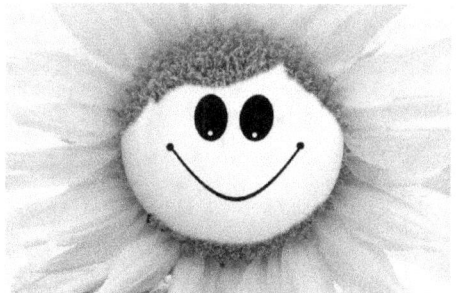

HAVE A NICE DAY!